Chemotherapy?
No thank you!

Part 1

The true story of my healing from breast cancer, lymphoma, bone and pleural metastases with without chemotherapy or any operations.

Inka Sattler

Disclaimer:

As the author is not a therapist, she expressly points out to her readers that this story should not encourage them to trifle with their illness. Furthermore, this book is no substitute for treatment from a capable therapist.

Translator: Hilary Teske

Copyright:

My heartfelt thanks go to
Hilary, without whom this book
would not have been possible.

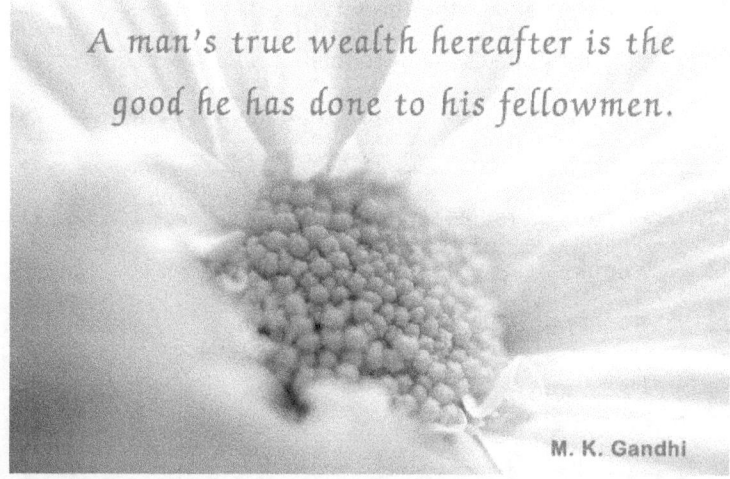

A man's true wealth hereafter is the
good he has done to his fellowmen.

M. K. Gandhi

Table of Contents

1. Preface

In the course of her life, Inka Sattler suffered from two different kinds of breast cancer, from lymph cancer and from bone cancer (involving paraplegia), from pleural cancer and leukaemia and two melanomas. The first incidence of cancer began in 2004 and the last ended in 2011. Seen from a purely statistical point of view, she would be dead with 300% probability today if she had decided on conventional medical treatment. At one point she was a case for nursing care at the highest level (3) and was lying in the palliative care unit. Today Inka, a keen horse-rider, has largely recovered and can carry out her tasks in life and even ride again cautiously. What is the basis for this miracle? While Inka was trying out about 20 alternative therapies during her illness, all of which proved to be more or less unsuccessful, useless and even harmful, when it came to the crux she always followed the findings of the "Germanic Medicine" (formerly "New Medicine") of the physician Dr Ryke Geerd Hamer (Norway).

This was her recipe for success, which not only several times saved Inka's life but also ensured that she has recovered her health today. Once the cancer diagnosis has hit them, most people do not have the strength to question the procedure prescribed by conventional medicine, let alone escape it.

With Inka, it was exactly the opposite – and that is the actual miracle. As she used to be a staff nurse, she knew what happened to breast cancer patients, refused to have the standard treatment (chemotherapy), found the Germanic Medicine and survived.

That is why her example is so important; for it shows that it is possible to follow the "New Medicine" successfully, when you have already been hit by the hammer of the conventional medical diagnosis – and get completely well again!

Here you can read how Inka managed to get well again.

2. The enemy in my body

I felt as if I was straight out of one of those glossy pharmacist's magazines "paid for by your pharmacist" (at that time I still believed that was correct, while today I know that the pharmaceutical industry of course uses the magazine to advertise and thus finances it, but the customer is not supposed to know that if possible and should think the pharmacist's magazine is an unbiased health guide).

I was standing under the shower and definitely not looking for any irregularities on my body – why should I have been? But there was something there and on one point the pharmacist's magazines were probably right in their advice. When you are soaping your body in the shower you are really most likely to find what nobody likes to find: I felt a lump in my right breast. At the beginning I tried to reassure myself by telling myself that the lump was certainly dependent on my menstrual cycle and would disappear again. I didn't think any more about it. But over time the small lump increased in size and I resorted to the remedies that had often helped both myself and my female relatives and friends (I have often been described as a "walking homeopathic encyclopaedia" because I have been educating myself on this subject for 25 years): so I applied a homeopathic ointment to my breast and also took homeopathic globules. I hoped that this would also work this time. But things were different: the lump grew incessantly and after a while it was even clearly to be seen externally through my T-shirt. And what was almost even worse was that an acute pain flashed through the affected breast like a stab from a knife from time to time, especially at night. The pain was so severe that it sometimes woke me up. Thus, I often lay awake at night during that time and felt completely helpless because of the pain in my breast and my fear of the "threat" from the "enemy in my body." Those nights I felt so dreadfully alone and in my despair and helplessness I wept my way through the sleepless nights with fervent prayers. I had not expected that! The reader will now wonder why I didn't say anything to my husband, a girl-friend or my mother. That is perhaps not so easy to understand: I didn't want my husband to panic and so didn't tell him about my worries for a long time. At the beginning, immediately after discovering the lump, I still hoped that it would disappear of itself. And when the lump had got so big that it visibly disfigured my breast, I had no more courage to tell my husband about it. After some time, I confided in a good friend, who initially reassured me. Oh, she had once had that, too!! Don't panic! It will go away again. But the lump didn't go away again! On the contrary, it grew and so did my panic. Was should I do? I was desperate and felt helpless and at the mercy of my fate.

Now I imagine my reader scratching their head and wondering why in the world I hadn't gone to the doctor long ago with the lump, which I had incidentally measured at that time. It was about 8x8 cm in size, very hard and coarse and protruded (under the – thank goodness – intact skin) so dominantly that at that time I wore padded bras so that nobody could see what my breast looked like. In addition, it was now getting increasingly difficult to "hide" my breast from my family.

In order to explain what prompted me NOT to go to the doctor, I have to take a brief look at the past, in my active time as a nurse.

3. My experience with chemo-toxins as a nurse

From that time in the hospital I still have vivid memories of what happened to patients who were admitted to the hospital with the diagnosis of a cancer tumour: they mostly arrived on the ward in a good general state but visibly discouraged. They were discouraged because of the cancer diagnosis; I didn't experience anybody who was not shocked by this. And we nurses and also the doctors put these patients in a quite specific way-of-no-return drawer, on which "CA patient" (Latin carcinoma = cancer) was written in invisible letters that could, however, be clearly seen by all of us (somewhere in this drawer the five phases of dying, which we had all learnt at one time in our training, even seemed to be waiting to be applied): we treated the poor patients with empathy during their last phase of life – with empathy especially because we constantly experienced that this diagnosis would sooner or later end in death for most of the patients.

At that time there was no palliative care unit but there was a palliative concept; however, first of all an examination was carried out and the doctors mostly found one or more "metastases" (secondary tumours) and then it was obligatory (with or without a finding of metastases) – chemotherapy had to be carried out fast!!! (There was no question about this being the only way to save the sick person, who was in a state of shock from the diagnosis, for the "aggressive" tumour would otherwise virtually devour the patient from inside. The doctors left the patient no time at all to think about the recommended therapy, for they put pressure on them by saying that if there was any delay in carrying out chemotherapy the metastases would spread through the body unhindered – and after all, nobody wanted that!

At the time when I worked in the hospital I was still very young (when I was 20 I was a fully trained nurse) and had been trained in conventional medicine. Thus, I had no fundamental doubts about what had been drummed into me for three years at nursing college. But I also strictly refused to prepare the chemotherapy for the patients. I didn't want to have anything to do with that poison. I was intuitively afraid... not necessarily for myself but for my unborn children. Nevertheless, I didn't of course know the conditions under which chemotherapy was prepared for the patient: the (poor) nurse stands in a full set of protective clothing in a tiled room and prepares the "beneficial" substance, naturally wearing a work coat, protective gloves and a surgical mask. At that time I was not aware that it was mustard gas from World War II (cf. Wikipedia). I only knew that it must be some kind of chemical toxin. It wasn't clear to me how and why that was then supposed to vanquish the cancer in the body and at the age of 20 I didn't think very much about it but (unfortunately) left the thinking to the doctors from conventional medicine, who would know about it. Only one thing was already branded into my memory: if ever I got into such a situation, i.e. if I should get cancer, I would not let such a toxin be administered to me. However, that wasn't clear to me from the start but the realisation only grew during the ten years I worked at the hospital.

4. Alone and in despair

One evening I was standing where it had all begun – under the hot shower. I was absolutely miserable about my now unsightly breast and was at a loss as to what to do. I don't know if I might have gone to the doctor after all if I hadn't been suffering from a considerable shift of day and night at that time. I didn't wake up until late afternoon and was then as a rule so busy with my daily tasks that I wouldn't have managed to go to a doctor. I didn't realise that was good until much later.

5. A lecture that changed my life

At that time I was still trying the ostrich method of hiding my head in the sand and still hoping at the same time that homeopathy, my prayers or something else would have an effect. But the opposite was the case. The lump wouldn't disappear. How much longer could I hide it from my family?

I thus carried my trouble around with me alone and prayed over my worries.

Then, one Saturday evening, I was reading the daily paper and an advertisement in bold letters in the events section absolutely struck me in the eye: "**This lecture will change your life**!" ... Today I know that it wasn't chance that I went there; it was my first lecture of that kind and it wasn't even in the direct vicinity of the place where I lived! I would say "it" attracted me magically. I was accompanied by my dear Mum; we found ourselves in a multi-purpose hall and didn't have any clue as to what was awaiting us!

The hall was quite full and I tried to guess what we had actually come to hear from the appearance of the other people in the audience. They were completely normal people like my Mum and me. Then the lecturer, a radiesthetist and alternative practitioner by profession, started to talk. What he had to say was really interesting: he spoke about living water, healthy and pathogenic salt, acidosis, earth radiation and how you can find it and – he said that cancer is curable in a completely natural way. Boom!! He simply said it as if he had said that the church bells ring in Bavaria in the morning: cancer is curable. I was so gobsmacked that I didn't catch anything of his explanation and that very thing disappointed me. There I was sitting with the lump in my breast, which to make matters worse was increasingly causing me stabbing pain, the man at the front seemingly had a solution – and I couldn't grasp it, couldn't follow it or whatever.

In the break we went to the tables with the items the lecturer was offering for sale, such as rods, mandalas, energy wands, pendulums and ... oh, what was that? There it was in bold letters: **C A N C E R**!!! – a booklet with the picture of a young woman with naked breasts for the price of one euro and I soon had it in my pocket (after paying for it, of course!). I must say that I would probably also have bought the booklet if it had cost 100 euros, so much did it appeal to me.

After the break, I couldn't get anything more out of the lecture as the booklet was making itself felt all the time from the depths of my handbag, wanting to be read at all cost. Perhaps it would explain exactly what the speaker had said about cancer healing itself!! After the lecture we drove home and I pulled the book, which seemed to have come right on cue, out of my handbag in great suspense – "Cancer and the five natural laws of a new biological medicine."

6. *Liberating knowledge at last: healing is possible!*

I got ready for bed and slipped under the quilt with the booklet. The Depesche about cancer thus became my bed mate that night. I naturally began reading in the hope that I would get information on how I could at last get rid of the lump in my breast. I became more and more enthralled with every page I read. I read about the German physician Dr Hamer and that due to his own cancer he had recognised in the 1980's why cancer develops at all. He called his discovery of the five biological laws the New Medicine (NM) and, among other things, formulated the "iron law of cancer" which says the following:

Every incidence of cancer and cancer-equivalent diseases develops due to a most severe, highly acute, dramatic and isolative conflict shock, which hits the individual completely unexpectedly like a crushing blow, virtually catching them "off guard." Dr Hamer called such a conflict experience shock a "Dirk Hamer syndrome," abbreviated as DHS.

This was explained very clearly in the little depesche with the example of a young mother standing at the side of the street when her child pulls away from her and gets under the screeching tyres of a passing car. The mother is hit by this incident completely unprepared (caught off guard), understandably experiences it as a severe shock and is left completely alone with her experience. She thus meets all the criteria of the iron rule of cancer and suffers a DHS in the moment she realises her child has been hit by a car. From this moment on, the mother is conflict-active, meaning that the conflict is persisting. The mother can only think of her sick child, she can hardly eat anything, can hardly sleep and has cold hands and feet. Dr Hamer therefore describes this conflict-active phase as the "cold phase," which lasts exactly until her child is well again. At the moment the DHS occurs, the mother's body reacts without reason on three levels: from the moment the DHS occurs, a "Hamer Herd" (HH) can be seen in the brain, a kind of "short-circuit" in the brain, in which nerve connections are torn. This impact is represented in a computer tomogram of the skull (or the brain) – which is what impressed me most on my first contact with the NM! – and a trained eye obtains information as to which phase of the disease the patient is in and which target organ is affected. On the physical level, the mother reacts with cell growth in her breast.

As already said, the mother's reaction is completely without reason; it has programmed itself into our cells for millions of years and still functions today as the significant biological special program (SBS) discovered by Dr Hamer.

Why is it called a significant biological special program? When you know, it is quite easy to comprehend it practically as the medical eureka. It may best be understood in a comparison: let's imagine a fawn is attacked by a wolf and injured. However, the wolf is disturbed in the act and so the little fawn survives and the mother, shocked by the wolf's attack, now needs more milk to enable the badly injured fawn to recover quickly. And exactly the same thing happens to the young mother in our example: due to the significant biological special program there is a proliferation of cells in the mother's mammary glands. This makes it possible for her breast to produce more milk and enables the injured child to get well as soon as possible. The moment the child is well again, the breast cancer caused by the growth of cells disintegrates – all by itself. That is part of the significant biological special program.

So far the story made sense to me: a growth of cells, which conventional medicine would clearly call "breast cancer" because of the fast-growing cells in the breast tissue, makes sense in a young mother who is greatly concerned about her baby.

However, it was still not clear to me how I could translate this new finding to my breast cancer.

7. Light at the end of the tunnel

So I devoured this Depesche and read it to the end in one go. Due to Mr Kent's (the author of the Depesche) personal way of explaining things simply, fast and precisely, after an hour I had the feeling that I could see light at the end of the tunnel. Over ten years have passed since that night but today I still know exactly how I felt after reading that Depesche: I had arrived in a different reality. The worry about my breast, with which I was completely alone, appeared in a totally new light. Could it be that everything is that simple?

My emotional world seemed to be reeling. What had been drummed into me during all those years of my training as a nurse and in my subsequent ten years of working as a nurse without my ever questioning it?

Cancer is a deadly disease that can only be fought in a few rare cases and exclusively with toxic chemotherapy, mutilating operations and life-threatening radiation. However, the malignant cancer cells mostly come back even after the use of "highly dosed chemotherapy" and the new highly praised "antibody therapies." Whereas, as already mentioned above, the patients were mostly flourishing before the devastating diagnosis of cancer, they were only a shadow of their former selves after the highly praised cancer treatments mandatorily prescribed in the doctors' guidelines. In the doctors' eyes (and also in the poor patients' eyes), the reason for the patients' extremely rapid physical and mental decline was never the aggressive therapies... no, no, no, the patients lost their hair because of the toxins (as it was always so nicely said: "No problem, your hair will grow again! And there are wigs as well!!"), they had diarrhoea and vomiting and many other "side-effects" (such nonsense that all undesired effects of medicines are called "side-effects" so as to make them seem harmless. However, these "side-effects" are in fact effects just as are the desired effects. There is no difference. Every medicine works as it works!) I felt sympathy for my patients when they visibly collapsed under the deadly treatment and I experienced how most of them went through hell. But the general decline of the poor cancer patients was naturally ascribed to the evildoer par excellence, the scourge of humanity, the cancer.

I have to honestly admit that I didn't realise either that not the cancer but the treatment could destroy people.

But everything in its turn. I hadn't yet actually gained that knowledge then. So I had read through the cancer Depesche in one go and was as if spellbound. WHO had given me this information now? Today I am still surprised at how I came to the Depesche through this "chance" but now I had it and while I was being painfully reminded of the massive lump in my breast by the "knife stabs," I thought: either this is the greatest humbug of all time... or... my SALVATION!!! I want to pre-empt things here: since that first Depesche night (up to today there have followed umpteen more Depesche days and nights with always new insights, but I think I can say that one cancer Depesche was not only the reason that I am writing this but also plays a part in my still being alive at all. I know that sounds exaggerated. But wait till the end of this article to judge if I have been exaggerating (-: ...

Where was I? Well, since that first Depesche night ten years ago I haven't found anything that is NOT correct in Dr Geerd Ryke Hamer's NM!

I don't want to neither can I explain the New Medicine here; Mr Kent's Depesche does that and other detailed literature as well.

But I would like to explain how I managed to recognise the cause of my unwanted lump with the help of the New Medicine.

In spite of the doubts my conventional medical conscience wanted to instil in me, I had had the feeling from the start that this would be the way I could get well again – without aggressive therapies. So I obtained further information to understand the overall picture. The greatest help was a study group near where I lived. There I was also able to acquire Dr Hamer's table, which was hot from the press at that time. I know exactly when I used it for the first time.

8. Recognising the cause of cancer

With the help of my study group leader, Hans, who has a huge amount of knowledge of the NM and supported me in a highly motivated and selfless way and got me out of my anxiety, I recognised the content of the conflict which had triggered my breast cancer: first of all, it was important to establish if I was right- or left-handed, for only then is it possible to ascertain whether the conflict which provoked the cancer had to do with the partner or with the mother-child side. I am right-handed, so the conflict must have had to do with a "partner" (in this case the partner can be either a life partner or a business partner or even a pet or some other friend or acquaintance), for my right breast was affected, i.e. the "partner breast." In addition, it was a cancer of the mammary ducts, which according to the NM means that the "partner was torn from my breast." It was a significant biological special program. What is meaningful about it? Nothing at all, from a rational point of view. But we all still have everything that used to be meaningful in our genes from our primal ancestors. When a (human or animal) child is "torn from its mother's breast," the mother's mammary ducts dilate as a result of the shock, which has the purpose that the milk which cannot be sucked in by the baby anymore doesn't drip out.

I reflected on what "partner" had been "torn from my breast" and it occurred to me spontaneously like scales falling from my eyes: a few months previously I had lost my greatly loved, faithful partner, who would have unhesitatingly fought with a lion just to prolong my life for a few seconds. Simba, my huge, jet-black cuddly Bernese mountain dog, who weighed 60 kilos and was as gentle as a lamb – THAT was it! I knew it at once as it was still burning in my soul that I had to have my dear doggy put to sleep prematurely and under highly dramatic circumstances. The liberating insight from this was that Dr Hamer was right!!

Now I was interested to see if my newly gained insight into the cause of my disease would be confirmed by my newly acquired scientific table compiled by Dr Hamer. For me it was vitally important to check if my "cancer" (I speak of cancer even if it is a significant biological special program, hereafter referred to as SBS) could be explained by natural laws and if I would find the conflict that had triggered my cancer.

I searched the table for "mammary tumour" (breast cancer) on the right side and was then rather disappointed: my supposition was not confirmed, for the table said that cancer of the right breast in a right-handed woman is assigned to a mother/child or mother/daughter conflict or a nest conflict. That was a bitter disappointment for me and led me to considerably doubt the insights into the five biological laws I had just gained. I had the feeling that my life would depend on whether the NM was right or not and so I immediately phoned Hans, my study group leader. He was also surprised, got out his table and rode the roller coaster for a moment: might it be that something had been confused in the table? The study group leader quickly regained confidence in his founded knowledge of the NM: it WAS a printing error! This luckily meant for me that the situation was just as we had worked out together. Now I was sure that my lump was the result of the loss of my dog, who had been "torn from my breast" in such a brutal and unplanned manner. I felt clearly that this was what had thrown me so off course.

It naturally made no sense from a rational point of view that my breast reacted to the dog which was torn from my breast. But every significant biological special program functions without reason. The body reacts in the same way it has been programmed to do in our cells for millions of years and it still functions like that today, whether we like it or not. And we have the choice of understanding and accepting it or fighting it with the weapons of conventional medicine, such as chemo-toxins, senseless operations and radiation – but unfortunately far too many lose this battle, for life itself – and a significant biological special program is nothing else – cannot be fought with anything in the world. The body doesn't make any mistake! I have relied on that since I recognised that the NM is right – and that was a good thing!

Ten years have now passed since I read the cancer Depesche. That time was different from today- I have heard from many cancer patients with whom I was recently in contact that they go on to the internet and just see what Google has to say on the subject of cancer. I didn't have that possibility then. That's why I am still all the more grateful today that fate played the cancer Depesche into my hands.

9. Healing in sight

So as not to bore the reader I will describe the continuation of my history in fast motion. When I was quite sure that the lump in my breast would not kill me because of my newly gained knowledge of the NM, I was glad at last to be able to tell my husband about what was going on in my body. First of all, I took every opportunity to inform him about the NM so that he would not panic when he heard about my lump. I managed that to a certain extent. It also took my husband a certain time to leave the accustomed path of conventional medicine and continue in the opposite direction. That was also badly needed as after a while the hot shower again confronted me with a fait accompli: I felt a lymph node the size of a chestnut in my right armpit, which must have grown overnight... my thoughts boiled hotter than the shower water for a moment, but then Hans, my study group leader, was suddenly with me in the shower. What did his sonorous voice always say in his lectures? Lymph nodes are also a sign of healing!!!" THAT was what I had been waiting for urgently and as crucial for my survival!! I quickly looked for Dr Hamer's table and made sure I had understood it properly. It was a load off my mind and off my husband's mind as well. Everything was all right: I was healing!! The main reason for this was our absolutely cute new puppy Cindy, who lovingly cuddled me over the loss of my unforgettable Simba.

During the time I got to know the NM, I contacted Dr Hamer and became acquainted with him as a loving, incomparable, fatherly and trustworthy doctor and person. He was so kind as to "read" my CCT (the scan of the layers of my brain) and was not only able to tell me which phase of the SBS I was in but could even read my whole life from the CCT as well. He saw a few other DHS's which had occurred in my life and which I was also able to confirm.

Dr Hamer was the one who always gave me courage again when my cares and pain repeatedly overwhelmed me. Thus, I decided to give others courage through my experience with breast cancer and gave Dr Hamer permission to publish my story in his book on breast cancer.

At that time I didn't think that I myself would write a book about my healing at a much later date.

10. Life sets its course

But life still had plenty in store for me.

Once my breast cancer or what conventional medicine considered to be breast cancer no longer caused my any difficulties, I got the medical diagnosis of osteolysis (bone cancer) of the vertebral column about four years later. One of my breast vertebrae had a pathological (i.e. resulting from a previous illness) multiple fracture and had caved in. There was an acute risk of my becoming paralysed from the waist down! I was in a state of shock. To my readers who are familiar with the NM and now cannot understand why I was shocked by this diagnosis, I say with due modesty that only someone who has had such a diagnosis can understand what it means for a person. Of course, (to my great fortune!!) I already knew the NM quite well at that time and I didn't doubt its correctness. But now something else besides my breast was affected: my backbone was BROKEN!

Once again Dr Hamer was our lifesaver! He took away our anxiety and supported us during the difficult time that followed. I would like to make it brief again: ten months after the shock diagnosis I was severely marked by the disease – paralysed from the waist down, totally emaciated and worn down by severe pain, I had to go to the palliative care unit because I had been losing more and more weight for months because of the strain of the pain and the paralysis and had to be fed parenterally (through a vein bypassing the digestive tract) in order to survive. I had become a "case for nursing care," completely dependent on outside help. I was not able to get out of bed for 18 months, not even in a wheelchair. The doctors described the computer tomography scans as "shattering:" my entire spine and pelvis were ridden with bone cancer. And if that was not enough, in addition I had a pleural tumour with an abscess and two melanomas the size of cherries were growing where the breast cancer had been: these finally burst so that I was lying there with a bleeding breast. Even Dr Hamer was concerned when he saw the CT scans and said flatly: "So there isn't much left…!"

The conventional doctors and nurses in the palliative care unit were a great help but also held a knife to my breast: with my "metastasising mammary carcinoma," as the official diagnosis termed it, I had no chance of living more than a few weeks if I did not at last agree to chemotherapy and an operation. It was simply incomprehensible to the doctors at the clinic that a person of my age could so radically refuse the treatment offered. It was not until four years later that I read in my report on discharge that the doctors assumed that I wanted "only palliative" treatment. In plain language, that means that they assumed I had given up hope. That was also the reason for the reproachful words of the doctor in charge of the unit: "Think about your children; they're still so young and need you!"

Because of my knowledge of the NM I refused the chemotherapy, antibody therapy, anti-hormonal therapy, operation and radiotherapy for my breast, which the doctors recommended, because I had decided to tackle the disease with the help of the biological laws discovered by Dr Hamer. Nothing was able to change my mind and that was a good thing.

In my book "Chemotherapy? No thank you! The miracle of my healing from cancer, metastases and paralysis" I have poured out my soul about how I managed to get back on my feet with God's help and my family's love, although the doctors had claimed that my legs would stay irreversibly paralysed.

In my book I write about over 20 of the sometimes risky therapies with which I more or less successfully accelerated my healing from cancer. The reader thus has help at hand to decide which of the treatments described come into question for them or their relatives and which are more or less a waste of time.

Here the New Medicine does not act as a therapy but a scientific foundation making healing possible at all.

To prevent misunderstandings I would like to make clear that three pillars carried me during the time I was ill: the first pillar was my family, which requires no explanations. The second pillar was my faith in the godhead above me and the third pillar was Dr Hamer's New Medicine. There might be confusion regarding the last two pillars. My faith helped me and I have a firm belief, but nevertheless it is a belief, as the word already says. And now comes the crucial thing: the NM has absolutely nothing to do with a belief. It is verified science in its purest form, as is unfortunately very frequently painfully missing in the dogmas strung together in our pseudo-scientific conventional medicine. Already on 8 and 9 September 1998 Dr Hamer was able to demonstrate and officially verify his five biological laws at the University of Trnava (Slovakia)! He could and would again provide evidence of his scientific findings to the medical fraternity of a German university at any time if they would only let him. However, the medical fraternity or rather the pharmaceutical lobby know what will happen when Dr Hamer's five biological laws are recognised: conventional medicine as it exists today will vanish from one day to the next. An exception is, of course, our emergency medicine, which renders outstanding services to patients. And what do our clever demi-gods in white do to avoid a confrontation with Dr Hamer on a medical level (because they know exactly that they cannot refute Dr Hamer's findings!)? They simply start legal proceedings against Dr Hamer. But what is Dr Hamer officially guilty of? Unfortunately people have also died in his care because they had already undergone a conventional medical pseudo-therapy before they contacted Dr Hamer: after chemotherapy, radiation and operation they were seen as "incurable" and were in an accordingly bad state. However, most of these patients survived in Dr Hamer's care – but not all of them. But because some 1,500 people also die of cancer (or chemotherapy) every day in conventional medicine alone in Germany, Dr Hamer could not be sentenced for not being able to save all his patients either. So a ruse was used and Dr Hamer was sentenced to imprisonment for treating patients when his licence to practice as a doctor had been withdrawn. And thus, to my great regret, Dr Hamer is today still a criminal sentenced by the German judiciary. He who deciphered a decisive part of the human code, thus revealing the scourge of humanity as a significant biological special program, as he calls the processes in the human body when a reaction takes place on a physical level and in the brain, has to flee from his beloved homeland because he is considered a wanted criminal in Germany.

On the other hand, the conventional doctors who are responsible for people dying from their deadly therapies every day because an effective cancer therapy is being suppressed, sun themselves in the light of their vanity and let themselves be celebrated as modern health professionals with Nobel prizes. As Dr Bruker so wisely said, no causal research is done in scientific medicine but pseudo-causes are invented.

Dr. med. M. O. Bruker, health doctor (1909-2001)

11. Free rider therapies

After my recovery from cancer of five organs I was repeatedly asked how I got well again. Everyone expected me to mention some special therapy, which I would then call the cancer therapy par excellence. But the basis of my recovery was Dr Hamer's NM. It is not a therapy but was the foundation of my healing that helped me the most of all ways of healing! As so far no name exists for this phenomenon, I have invented one; it was literally forced upon me that a name is needed for therapies that – mostly more or less by chance – take place simultaneously with the body's biological healing phase (for example, hyperthermia, special therapies with diets, supplements or vitamins, innumerable miracle herbs for cancer and rituals for curing cancer or costly miracle healings which are assigned cancer-healing powers), which, however, have no connection with the cause of healing. The name I have invented is free rider therapies. Read more about it in my book.

12. My book

> „Chemotherapy? No thank you! Part 2
> The miracle of my healing from cancer,
> metastases and paralysis."

During the two years of my illness, I again and again made notes about the course of my illness and the good and not so good events at that time. And in this way my "diary of healing from cancer" has become a book about how cancer is biologically curable. However, it makes absolute sense to read this book BEFORE you fall into the well or before you get cancer, just as it is known to be advisable to learn to swim before you fall into the water.

Here is an explanation of the title of the book "Chemotherapy? No thank you! The miracle of my healing from cancer, metastases and paralysis." I thought for a long time about what I should call my book. For people familiar with the NM the title would have been "How I got through the healing crises of five (if we count the lymph node in my armpit and the leukaemia it was seven) SBS's with the help of the NM." But people who have not yet heard of the NM would not have connected this title with the subject of "cancer" at all.

I have to admit that I myself was not able to identify with the title of my book initially. But a very large number of people who experienced how I was nearer to death than life during my illness and now experience me four years after the low point of my illness have said again and again: "THERE a miracle happened!" and even for people familiar with the NM this story of disease is probably not so commonplace.

So I think I can say in all modesty that the title of my book is not too bold. I very much hope that my book manages to accomplish what I have written it for: it is intended to encourage people to trust in the self-healing powers of their own bodies. Our body has been so brilliantly created; it never makes a mistake. And that is why it is quite certain that cancer is biologically curable!

My book: *Chemotherapy? No thanks Part 2: The miracle of my healing from cancer, metastases and paralysis* is available from Amazon.com

13. Summary of the book:

This autobiographical story recounts the dramatic experiences of 47-year-old Inka Sattler, who with the diagnosis "Exulcerated mammary tumour with diffuse osseous and pleural metastases" (in plain English: "Burst breast cancer with bone and pleural metastases") finds herself paralysed from the waist down in the palliative care unit. There the doctors predict that she will only live a few more weeks and will never be able to walk again. This book has been written five years after the initial diagnosis: her breast has long since healed and Inka, a former staff nurse, can walk again. And this happened although (or just because!!!) she refused to have the recommended chemotherapy, antibody therapy, antihormonal therapy or any operations. In this very personal account, written from her soul, she describes how she managed to let her body heal.

Over 20 of the sometimes risky therapies which Inka underwent to more or less accelerate her healing from cancer are described. The reader is thus given help in deciding which of the treatments presented come into question for themselves or their relatives.

In this way the "diary of healing from cancer" has become a book about how cancer is biologically curable. However, it makes absolute sense to read this book BEFORE you fall into the well or before you get cancer, just as it is known to be advisable to learn to swim before you fall into the water. The net proceeds from this book are donated to social causes.

http://www.amazon.com/Chemotherapy-No-thanks Part 2-miracle-metastases/dp/1519217684/ref=sr_1_fkmr0_1?ie=UTF8&qid=1452552192&sr=8-1-fkmr0&keywords=chemotherapy+no+thank+you

The photo on the back cover shows Inka Sattler, as she comes slowly back on to her feet after her cancer and paralysis.

www.ingramcontent.com/pod-product-compliance
Lightning Source LLC
Chambersburg PA
CBHW061238180526
45170CB00003B/1345